CONTENTS

INTRODUCTION

Mental health is such an important topic to talk about. Amy Morin is a psychotherapist, mental strength trainer, and international bestselling author. With over 15 million views, her TED Talk "The Secret of Becoming Mentally Strong" is one of the most popular talks of all time. Additionally, Amy Morin has dedicated her career to studying the habits of mentally strong people.

"So I have a Facebook friend who's life seems perfect….How many of you have a friend kind of like that and how many of you don't like that person sometimes?"

Amy Morin, "The Secret of Becoming Mentally Strong," TEDxOcala (2015).

The auditorium responds to this question with laughter, as this is one of the first things Amy Morin says in her inspirational speech. However, the widespread laughter stopped as Morin began to express how this way of thinking costs us our mental strength.

Amy Morin goes on to explain the traps our minds set for us to eventually fall into bad habits. Moreover, she discusses the three most common unhealthy habits we happen to fall into, the ways we can change our actions, and ultimately–how to begin this process.

Eventually, Morin goes into detail on the unhealthy habits and beliefs that keep us from being mentally strong and moreover, shares her own story. In doing so, Morin stresses that you need to be prepared to give up bad beliefs because you cannot afford not to.

"There comes a time when we need all the mental strength you can muster."

If you are interested in reading more about this incredible TED Talk and Amy Morin's advice, keep reading:

◆ ◆ ◆

A Brief Background On Amy Morin

Amy Morin is editor-in-chief at VeryWell Mind, a licensed clinical social worker, psychotherapist, and psychology lecturer at Northeastern University. Morin has written four books. Her most recent book, *13 Things Strong Kids Do*, went on sale in April of this year. It is geared toward kids from ages 8-12 and teaches them mental strength exercises to enhance their childhood and help them transition into becoming a teenager.

Morin regularly writes articles for Forbes, Business Insider, and Psychology Today, where over 2 million people devour her content on mental strength each month. The Guardian named her as "The self-help guru of the moment," while Forbes called her a "leadership star."

Amy Morin received her bachelor's degree in social work from the

University of Maine and her master's in social work from the University of New England.

She also is the host of the Verywell Mind podcast for mentally strong people, where she interviews guest speakers from around the world about their successes and struggles. The podcast launched in September of last year and can be found across all major streaming sites. Morin can be found relaxing on a sailboat in the Florida Keys, which also doubles as her podcast studio.

AMY MORIN: HER STORY

At the young age of 23, Morin had just graduated from graduate school. Amy was just starting her career, getting married, and even moving into a new home. However, Morin was devastated to learn of her mother's passing from a brain aneurysm. Amy expressed how she pitied herself for years, and, like most of us would–she wondered why she had to lose her mother so soon. She assumed that her mother would be around for many more years to come.

Amy Morin gave herself time to grieve for her mother, and after some time, Morin felt like the feeling in the pit of her stomach was starting to lessen. On the three-year anniversary of her mother's death, Amy and her husband Lincoln were invited to attend a basketball game. Consequently, the event was held at the very same place Morin had last seen her mother prior to her death. However, Amy and Lincoln still decided to go.

Afterwards, Lincoln was admitted into the hospital. Amy's husband ultimately passed away from a heart attack. Once again, Morin fell into grief over another shocking, unthinkable loss.

The self-pity was all consuming and Amy found her-

self wondering, "I'm a 26-year-old widow without a mom...What am I to do?"

Still, Amy Morin took the necessary steps to try and avoid falling into a bad mindset. Four years later, Amy had met her new husband, Steve. As she settled into her life, she grew close to her new father-in-law. In yet another tragedy, her father figure was diagnosed with inoperable cancer, and Amy once again lost someone she loved.

"Why is this happening to me again?"

Somehow, Morin challenged herself to identify all the unhealthy habits she would avoid during her grief. Eventually, Amy came to the conclusion that building mental strength required understanding destructive beliefs.

DESTRUCTIVE BELIEFS

In her infamous TED Talk, Morin explains that bad habits, thoughts, and beliefs are costing you more than you realize. She takes us back to her introduction, where we laughed over disliking a Facebook friend who seems to have a 'perfect' life. Researchers have found that envying your friends on Facebook can lead to depression. In fact, even feeling envious for 5 seconds is taking away too much time from focusing on yourself.

"Establishing healthy habits–like eating a healthy diet, getting plenty of sleep, and participating in regular exercise–can also go a long way to improving how you feel."

Morin divides these destructive beliefs into three categories. This way of thinking, Amy believes, robs you of much needed mental strength.

Unhealthy Beliefs About Ourselves

The first of these destructive beliefs stems from being uncomfortable with feelings. In these cases, you find yourself feeling sorry for yourself. While it is normal to feel sad, you are only magnifying that misfortune by saying things like: "Why do things like this always happen to me?"

Lying in this self-pity is only a temporary distraction from the pain. These thoughts about ourselves keep us stuck in a bad mindset, and you are only focusing on the problem. That is, you are not thinking about ways to heal. The solution is to go through the pain, allow yourself to feel those emotions fully, and then you can begin to move on.

Unhealthy Beliefs About Others

Another bad habit is thinking that other people control us, and, as a result, we give them our power. These sorts of destructive beliefs come out when we say things like: "My mother-in-law is such a pain." The truth is, we live in a free world, and there are very few things that we have to do.

"Your thoughts greatly influence how you feel and behave. In fact, your inner monologue has a tendency to become a self-fulfilling prophecy."

In other words, you are always in control of how you react to others around you. Letting your mother-in-law or even your boss affect you or your mood is your choice; holding onto that reaction only means holding yourself back. The best solution is to only compare yourself to the person you were yesterday–never anyone else.

Unhealthy Beliefs About The World

The final destructive belief stems from this general idea that the world is a fair place. In reality, good actions aren't always rewarded. For another example, people often say "hard work guarantees success." Maybe this is true for some people, but it is just not the way the world works. The world is what you make of it, but you have to change your own thoughts first. Start to accept things around you (even the negative things) so you can prepare for disappointment and how to move on.

"Mental strength is like physical strength; you have to cut out the junk food."

In other words, you have to give up the bad habits and start exercising the good ones. Train your brain to give up the bad mental habits. For example, you can trade out resenting someone's success with practicing gratitude for all the good things you have in your life.

◆ ◆ ◆

One Small Step

If there is anything to take away from Amy Morin's speech, it's that one change can make a big difference. In fact, sometimes taking the first step is just what you need. Training your mind is a domino effect; once you have a solid, positive perspective–so many of your actions will change.

Amy Morin illustrates this concept through speaking about her encounter with a man who has diabetes. Morin tells the audience how this man's diabetes was genetic, and it was passed down from his mother. As a result, the man believes his life is doomed, and he decides not to make any changes to his diet or exercise. Eventually, the man loses his vision license without making these changes.

"While ignoring your bad habits may help you feel good initially, that avoidance will eventually catch up to you. When you don't address the unproductive and unhealthy things you're doing alongside your good habits, you'll stagnate."

Although he knew he could do something to change his situation, he didn't think making the changes would be worth it. In the end, Morin shares, the man decides to swap regular soda for diet soda and his numbers changed drastically. After this, the man decided to make goals to get his vision back; and he had a specific goal in mind to reach it. It is easy to see how one small step can change your mindset, and how a changed mindset can affect your life.

WHAT THE MENTALLY STRONG DON'T DO

Amy Morin's bestselling book, "13 Things Mentally Strong People Don't Do" highlights some of the most common bad habits that hold people back from living a full and rich life. Whether you are training to become a brain surgeon or working on becoming a more attentive partner, mental strength will come in handy for both situations despite how different they appear to be.

No matter what your goals are, building up your mental strength will help toward achieving those dreams. Learning to pinpoint the pitfalls that you are most prone to can help send you on your way to turning into your best self.

Here are the 13 things that Amy Morin says mentally strong people don't do:

Waste Time Feeling Sorry For Themselves

A lot of life's inconveniences, setbacks, and sorrows are inevitable, but feeling sorry for yourself won't get you anywhere or fix your problems. Every single person in the world is dealing with some type of struggle or loss. Yes, even rich people such as Kylie Jenner, who seems to have it all, endures some type of hardship.

Whether you are barely scraping by and struggling to make ends meet, going through a messy breakup, or dealing with a loved one's newly diagnosed health issues, wallowing in self-pity won't alleviate the pain. In fact, it only works to enhance it and serve as a reminder of your misfortunes.

If you tend to indulge in self-pity when sorry situations arise in your life, train your brain to replace self-pity with gratitude. Focus on how much you already have rather than what you've lost. Mentally strong people don't waste their valuable time and energy thinking about their problems and completely drowning in emotion. Once your time is gone, there's no getting it back. Instead, they concentrate their attention on coming up with a solution.

Give Up All Of Their Power

This habit falls under one of the categories of destructive beliefs, which is the second one: unhealthy beliefs about others. People who give up their power do so by blaming others for their problems or when things go downhill. As mentioned previously, letting your mother-in-law or your boss upset you gives them control over you.

"...allowing a negative person to dictate your emotions gives them too much power in your life. Make a conscious effort to choose your attitude."

If you think about them in a negative light, the effect this will have on your mood and behavior will be negative as well. You cannot blame them for the way you feel because you have the ability to choose how you respond to them.

In order to take back your power, you must accept responsibility for how you think, behave, and feel. This is essential toward building your mental strength and leading a more meaningful life.

Avoiding Change

Change is a natural part of life, but many people absolutely dread it, or even fear it. If things never changed, we would fail to grow and just stay stuck in the same place for the rest of our lives. That's why change is good. It makes us better. So then, why do so many of us go out of our way to avoid change? This is because change is uncomfortable. Instead of embracing change, we prefer to shy away from new challenges and stick with what's familiar to us.

Learning to recognize when you avoid change, like turning down a job offer, refusing to leave an unhealthy relationship, or even something as simple as incorporating different foods into your diet, can lead toward a new and improved life. It takes practice to become accustomed to the feeling of discomfort that comes along with change, but once you learn how to tolerate it, your confidence in the ability to forge your own path will grow.

Waste Energy On Things They Can't Control

The cold, hard truth is that you do not have control over many of the events that occur in life. Worrying about things we can't control only serves to pile on more unnecessary stress. The state of the economy and the decisions that other people make are just a few examples of things that can't be controlled. Agonizing over them will only disturb your peace and deplete you of the mental strength you need to be your best self.

The sooner we are able to accept the truth, the quicker we can get on our way to actual productivity. Some people who fight the facts of life become total control freaks. They believe that if they can gain enough control over people, they can keep bad things from happening. This can also lead to other toxic habits, such as micromanaging and picking apart other people's choices, therefore effectively ruining relationships.

"Wasting brain power ruminating about things you can't control drains mental energy quickly. The more you think about problems you can't solve, the less energy you'll have leftover for more productive endeavors."

You can't stop a storm from coming, but you can prepare yourself for it. Determine what you can do, and focus on that instead. Not only will it distract your mind from inevitable circumstances, but it will also be beneficial towards your well-being.

Worry About Pleasing Others

It's hard not to care about what others think of you because nobody wants to experience feelings of hurt and rejection when someone disapproves of you. People pleasers generally have low self-esteem and their self-worth is derived from other people's approval. This causes them to sabotage their own goals to fulfill the satisfaction of others. Constantly trying to please others and avoid conflict at all costs is not healthy and can result in depression.

Doing your own thing and saying what you truly think takes a lot of courage. It is tempting to agree with the popular opinion to make yourself look good. However, in order to stay true to yourself and live an authentic life, you must stick to your own values and refuse to bend to others' will, even when your beliefs or choices are not the standard. It may feel distressing at first to go against the grain, but you'll be happier overall in the long run.

"Your words and your behavior must be in line with your beliefs before you can begin to enjoy a truly authentic life. When you stop worrying about pleasing everyone...you'll experience many benefits."

Fear Risk-taking

If you stop to think about it, you will realize that we make hundreds of choices, both big and small, every single day without really considering the risks behind them. Whether it's getting behind the wheel of a car or investing in the stock market, emotions often play a part in the choices we make. If you feel afraid, your decision may be clouded by paranoia and uncertainty, possibly extending the amount of time it takes for you to decide on anything. Fear does not let you accurately measure the levels of risk in a decision, and it can even go so far as to prevent you from making the best choices. Learning how to set your emotions aside will allow you to see each option more clearly. Then, your selection will be chosen based on careful calculations rather than senseless emotion.

Dwell On The Past

After something stressful happens where we feel like we might have made the wrong decision, it would be nice if we could just leave it behind and forget all about the matter. At times, this can be done quite successfully, like when you receive a bad score on a test, you might feel down about it for a minute, and then just shake it off and move on to studying for the next upcoming exam. However, we more often than not, tend to continue to overthink and obsess over stressful events, especially when it's a fight with a significant other or a job interview at a prestigious company.

While reflecting on the past and learning from your mistakes can be helpful in determining what you can do better the next time around, rumination is what drags people down and causes them to sabotage their present and their future. These thoughts are not about active problem-solving, but about obsessions and anxieties. This is a huge issue because it robs you of the opportunity to enjoy yourself and live in the moment. Additionally, surrounding yourself with the familiarity of the past fuels a fear of the unknown future and contributes to persistent negative thinking.

Dwelling on the past is the biggest barrier from moving forward, and life will continue on whether you are ready or not. It also prohibits you from building mental strength. Making peace with the past and accepting past decisions will help you work toward endurance and becoming mentally strong.

Make The Same Mistakes

Sometimes it's simply not enough to make a mistake one time to avoid repeating it again forever. The larger majority of us are prone to repeating the same mistakes occasionally, and that's normal. The problem arises when you fail to own up to your faults and refuse to change your patterns. You cannot repeat the same mistakes and expect different results. That's just not the way it works. Simply vowing to never make the same mistake again is not the right approach because it is nothing but an empty promise that's standing in between you and the mistake.

Mentally strong people do not try to cover up their mistakes, instead they use them as opportunities to grow and acquire new knowledge. Learning from mistakes compels you to put time and energy into developing new strategies to minimize those mistakes. It also calls for you to trace the route of your decision making that brought you to the mistake in the first place. If you do not learn from your errors, they will become regrets.

"Sticking to good habits can be hard work, and mistakes are part of the process. Don't declare failure simply because you messed up or because you're having trouble reaching your goals. Instead, use your mistakes as opportunities to grow stronger and become better."

Hate Others For Their Success

People strive for success not just to obtain happiness or a higher salary, but to prove their worth to the world and to themselves. That's why you might feel resentful toward the co-worker who's receiving a promotion or your friend who's getting married before you. In our minds, it means that those successful people are more worthy and valuable than us. Hating other people for their success will get in the way of your own ability to reach your goals.

It seems important to mention that everyone's definition of success looks slightly different, which is why comparing yourself to others is damaging. It simply does not work; it's like comparing apples to oranges. Especially during the age of technology and social media, it has become more and more difficult to refrain from making comparisons.

Pay attention to when your thoughts revert to jealousy over someone's incredible bikini body or luxurious new car. Rather than pining after their achievements, remind yourself of how lucky you are and be proud of what you've accomplished. Once you have determined what your personal idea of success is, you'll actually start to become genuinely happy for other people's prosperities and be more committed to making your own dreams come true.

Give Up After Failure

There are quite a few jokes out there about people who give up on something after not being perfect at it on the first try. While these are merely jokes, the truth is embedded at its core and lurks closer to the surface than most people seem to realize. Many people actually give up on things far too quickly. After a few too many failures, we respond by quitting. If this is your answer to defeat, you are ensuring that you will never reach success. It is perfectly normal to feel embarrassed, discouraged, or be in low spirits when your first attempts don't go your way. Kids are taught at a young age that failure is a bad thing, causing them to look at failure in a negative light further down the road. But it is impossible to have success without failure. The two come hand in hand.

When you decide not to give up, you learn that there are hidden strengths and potentials within you that you never would've discovered if you hadn't kept moving forward. You also learn how to maintain your motivation. It is best to focus on thinking positive thoughts like, "I am capable of trying again," and to stop thinking untrue phrases like, "I can't do this."

Mentally strong people view the obstacles they face as evidence that they are working to the best of their abilities, pushing themselves to the limit, and generally doing all they can to advance further.

Avoid Alone Time

Many people avoid silence and solitude because it makes them feel uncomfortable. Spending time by yourself out in public is also something that is fervently avoided. People often associate being alone with boredom, sadness, and a variety of other negative feelings. Psychotherapist Karen R. Koenig says that:

"People often fear being alone because they are uncomfortable with their thoughts...They like being out with others or keeping busy because interaction and activity keep distressing thoughts at bay."

The fear of being alone may force you to continue staying in unhappy and unhealthy relationships. You may even be tempted to resort to scrolling through social media, which is not the answer. In fact, it might make you feel even worse. Although platforms such as Facebook, Instagram, and Twitter are meant to help you stay connected with people you don't see every day, spending too much time on those apps can further disconnect you from yourself.

Having time to yourself is a critical part of building mental strength. Create opportunities for some quiet time to be alone with your thoughts, reflect on life, and establish new goals for the future.

Feel A Sense Of Entitlement

Feeling a sense of entitlement toward a certain job, a person, or whatever else, will have you rooted to the same place for years because unfortunately, the world doesn't really owe you anything. If you're busy waiting for something good to come to you, you will let other opportunities pass you by–opportunities that could have helped you evolve and flourish.

Entitled people believe they are better than everyone else, and therefore deserve much more, when in reality, they are not as special as they think they are. According to researchers from Case Western University, entitlement typically leads to chronic disappointment because you never receive the things you believe you deserve, so you are constantly left with unmet expectations. If you feel a sense of entitlement, it is crucial to recognize how it is partly responsible for your downfall and lack of success.

Expect Immediate Results

In today's fast-paced world, we have grown so used to instant gratification in the form of text messages, Amazon delivery's two-day shipping guarantee, fast food drive-thrus, and numerous other things that our brains are becoming wired to believe that everything should happen in an instant. As a collective society, our patience is wearing thin.

It is important to keep in mind that unlike our order of a new pair of leggings, self-growth does not arrive in under 48 hours. It develops very slowly, but don't let that deter you from more meaningful pursuits. Slow and steady always wins the race and expecting immediate results will only lead to major disappointment.

Whether you're trying to lose a certain amount of weight or learn a new language, remember that true change does not happen overnight as we might expect it to. Pay attention to when you start to become irritated at the pace you're moving in your career, relationships, etc. There is no such thing as too slow or being behind in the circle of life. Even developing a stronger patience for smaller things such as your Starbucks order taking longer than usual can contribute to building mental strength.

"Mentally strong people don't shy away from change - nor do they expect immediate results."

Everyone has the ability to develop mental strength and to curb bad habits. However, in order to do so, it is necessary to come to an acute awareness of any self-destructive habits you might possess that are holding you back from living your best life. Once you recognize how any of the 13 habits might play a role in your life, you'll be able to work on becoming stronger and healthier in more ways than one.

WHAT MENTALLY STRONG WOMEN DON'T DO

You've read about what mentally strong people don't do. Now, get ready for Morin's additional advice from her other bestselling book, "13 Things Mentally Strong Women Don't Do." As mentioned in the title, this book focuses on the patterns of women. While all kinds of people can have the same bad habits, gender can play a huge role in what keeps you stuck in a rut or slows down your progress. Morin lays out the bad habits that women are more likely to engage in due to societal expectations, patriarchy, and gender bias.

Here are the 13 things that mentally strong women don't do:

Compare Themselves To Other People

You will not gain a single thing by measuring your happiness, appearance, wealth, and possessions with other people. That will only serve to drain you of your mental strength. Morin says that the only person you should compare yourself to is the person you were yesterday. Comparing yourself to others allows them to drive your behavior. When we compare ourselves to others, we are usually comparing their best features with our worst qualities or our most average ones. It's like being right-handed and trying to write with your left hand.

Sometimes, comparisons can be motivating but more often than not, they are destructive. You could work yourself to the bone trying to outscore the top student in the class, and the biggest thing you will have achieved is the destruction of your mental health. There will always be one thing that you are better at than anyone else, and that thing is being yourself. When you embrace this mindset, the world starts to look more hopeful again. You will become happier and free from the shackles of your own negativity. When focusing internally, you will find that the most important things in life come from the inside, not the outside.

"When you give up comparing yourself to other people you'll be free to focus on your best effort."

Women are taught to be spiteful, to view other women as competitors, and to constantly be vying for the attention of men. There's also a huge emphasis on beauty for women. We should always be looking our best, with not a hair out of place or a blemish in sight. Society always pits us against one another, so it's no surprise that this first habit on the list is one that we seem to struggle with most. It's been ingrained in us as a way to keep men on top and women to stay submissive. It will take a lot of discipline, determination, and hard work to shift that mindset. Cutting down on this kind of behavior will not only make you a better, healthier person, but it will inspire other women to do the same and empower women as a whole.

Insist On Perfection

Nobody is perfect, no matter how much we trick ourselves into believing otherwise. Perfectionism may feel like something to brag about; the term itself paints the picture of a hard working person who delivers high quality results. What you may not realize is that perfectionism holds you back from your full potential and can cause you to perform worse. The fear of making mistakes and not being good enough can be detrimental to your health.

Women are more likely to be perfectionists than men. This can be seen in various forms: applying for a new job, hesitating on asking for a promotion, and holding back from answering a question unless we are absolutely certain that our answer is correct. There is a pretty well known statistic circulating out there that states that men apply for a job when they meet only 60 percent of the qualifications while women only apply if they meet 100 percent. According to LinkedIn behavioral data, women opt themselves out if they do not meet all the criteria and end up applying to 20 percent less jobs than men.

Rather than crossing off an intriguing position from the list if you lack a couple of desired skills, widen your net and apply to jobs that interest you regardless of title or level. This strategy can be practiced in other areas of life as well. It helps to push your limits, broaden your horizons, and expand opportunities.

Perfectionists tend to set the bar incredibly high for themselves. Establishing high expectations is good, but too high of standards can leave you feeling useless. We are not superhuman. As you've probably heard countless times, failure is perfectly fine and it's a necessary part of life. Accept the fact that mistakes are part of the learning process and that you do not need to fulfill every standard out there to be considered good enough.

See Vulnerability As A Weakness

Asking for help, acknowledging your flaws, and admitting that you're struggling are often seen as signs of weakness when in reality, they are signs of strength. It takes courage to knowingly put yourself in a position where you risk being burned. Even Morin herself admits that it's not easy to expose your personal self to the outside world.

"Vulnerability is the last thing I want you to see in me, but the first thing I look for in you."

Vulnerability can be the key to forming healthier, happier, and more meaningful relationships. Those who keep vulnerability at bay to protect themselves from getting hurt oftentimes wind up missing out on close, intimate relationships. They waste too much time and energy hiding behind a facade and trying to please others.

Your association with vulnerability depends on your level of awareness of how much vulnerability can actually benefit you. Vulnerability can be shown in many ways like, saying "I love you" to someone for the first time or asking a question that might initially feel embarrassing. Putting up a front and erecting a wall around yourself prevents others from getting to know your true nature. You must accept your vulnerability if you wish to live a fuller and richer life. Even the simplest act of letting down your guard bit by bit helps with personal growth.

Let Self-Doubt Stop Them

Everyone has experienced episodes of self-doubt at one time or another. As women, we spend much of our lives wrestling with self-doubt, especially since society is not the greatest at uplifting women. But we don't have to let it stop us from pushing forward and reaching our goals. Don't listen to your brain when it's trying to tell you that you're not capable or not smart enough.

Some levels of self-doubt can actually be healthy; after all, it exists as a tool of safety to help keep us in check and notice when we are wrong or when something is too far out of our reach. Morin encourages us to let self-doubt fuel our effort. If we think we're going to fail at something, then naturally, we will work harder and put in more effort. In this manner, we can combat self-doubt and maybe even prove ourselves wrong along the way.

However, there are times when our self-doubt causes us to stand in our own way and makes it hard for us to see the good qualities in ourselves. This leads to insecurity about the sufficiency of our skills and we question our ability to confront new challenges. Morin also describes what else self-doubt can lead to, and none of them are very pleasant: an inability to tolerate the unknown, a greater need for validation, lower self-esteem, and of course, the two big culprits, anxiety and depression.

"The emphasis on achievement also plays into self-doubt. It sounds inspiring to tell girls that they can be anything they want, but unless we tell them how to deal with mistakes, failures, and setbacks, we're not giving them the skills they need to succeed."

Mentally strong women don't let self-doubt crush their confidence. They embrace a little self-doubt and use it to their advantage. They can also distinguish between when self-doubt is seeping in for sabotage and when self-doubt is being rational. It's easy to spot the difference when it's not your experience that you're looking at. One way to tell is when you notice yourself replaying negative past experiences over and over to justify not doing something in the present. When self-doubt creeps into your head, remind yourself that you can still succeed even if you're feeling low in confidence.

Overthink Everything

If you have a hyperactive imagination, you might find your mind wandering to images of the end of the world and other post-apocalyptic scenarios. This may cause you to spiral and panic about what you would do in that particular situation. If this sounds like you, remember that your thoughts are not predictions of the future. Overthinking includes two destructive thought patterns: ruminating and incessant worrying. It involves rehashing things from the past and negative thinking about the future. Overthinking means dwelling on your problems, not actually solving them.

"We don't know what life would have had in store for us had we not made those choices. But it's easy for us to imagine that life could be better if we could only change the past."

Overthinkers tend to ask for advice from anyone sympathetic enough to listen, although they do not truly listen to the advice doled out to them. Overthinking makes life harder than it needs to be. It wears down your resilience and even interferes with your sleep. Releasing yourself from the belief that excessive worry will protect you from harm or help you be prepared for disaster can be liberating.

A big takeaway from realizing that you are an overthinker is that your thoughts can consume you. But they don't need to. Pay more attention to the happy parts of your life and consider brighter possibilities of the future rather than scary ones. Think about what you are able to control and focus on that by engaging in problem solving and productive action.

Avoid Challenges

Whether it's getting back into your exercise routine, having an uncomfortable conversation with a friend, cleaning out the attic, or doing taxes, avoiding challenges will keep you stuck on the same track. We're always avoiding some difficult thing one way or another. Constantly checking our messages and notifications is the most common distraction we turn to when we're trying not to think about something.

Avoidance merely serves as a temporary relief from discomfort, pain, and difficulty. But if we never directly face the challenges in front of us or the turmoil going on inside of us, this means that we are at the mercy of our fears. You have to face challenges no matter what because tough stuff is always popping up in life. The longer you wait and put them off, the harder they are to overcome. Face your fears one baby step at a time and you will build the confidence and mental strength needed to tackle challenges. It won't happen overnight, but you'll get better at dealing with discomfort and refraining from procrastinating.

Never Break The Rules

Breaking the rules gives off a negative connotation and is often seen as a bad thing, but it can open a lot of doors if you're doing it with purposeful intentions and to take a stand. This is not to say that you should violate the law, disrespect others, and put people in harm's way or anything like that, but certain rules can sometimes trap us. Girls are encouraged early on in life to be polite and well-behaved while it's more acceptable for boys to get into mischief and stir up trouble. Morin says that women apologize more because they have a lower threshold for wrongdoing than men do. They feel compelled to follow the rules.

In a Q&A session conducted by Laura Connolly (Lauroly) from the blog World Wise Beauty, Morin talks about how women are taught to be compliant, but breaking the rules sometimes is necessary to incite change. She shares an example in her book about a woman who didn't stick to the norm. In 1967, Katherine Switzer became the first woman to complete a marathon. Up until then, women were not considered to be physically capable of running such a long distance. Switzer ran the race and proved to the world that women can run marathons. If she had not gone against the preconceived notion that women aren't strong, women would be even further behind in the sports industry today.

According to a 40-year study done by *Developmental Psychology*, kids who broke the rules were more likely to be higher earners as adults. With this in mind, let yourself break free from the unwritten rules of societal expectations and gender norms because they are meant to hold women back. Unlearn the limitations you were taught as a child, and instead, teach yourself that it is okay to be unconventional. That is how you'll be able to change the world. If women never broke the rules, we would not see much progress in society. Now, we have women in all industries working alongside men.

Whenever you might be wary about crossing the line, keep in mind that breaking a few rules can give you the satisfaction of knowing that you're the one with the biggest say over your own life. Even though some people will not be too thrilled with your decisions, you can gather strength from the fact that you stay true to yourself and stick to your own values and beliefs.

Lift Themselves Up By Putting Others Down

In a society rampant with competition and run by capitalism, the poisonous act of putting others down in order to lift oneself up, is becoming more and more apparent. This also stems from other things as well, like bullying, the need to feel superior, or an abusive home life. Because so many people do it nowadays, it might be tempting to jump on the bandwagon to get to the top. However, no one truly gets ahead by making others look bad and pointing out their faults. Even if you got to the top this way, you will only be uprooted from your position later by someone else drawing attention to your flaws and striving to drag you down.

No matter the situation, you can only control your own performance and make yourself better. You can't make other people worse. Putting energy into wanting others to fail takes the focus off of yourself and makes you drive off the road to success. When you lift others up and become a genuine cheerleader, you will receive support and encouragement from others in return. Your success will be more likely to stick around permanently. Mentally strong women don't see other women as their enemies. They look at the bigger picture and adopt the mindset that one woman's success is a win for all women.

"Be the woman who fixes another woman's crown without telling the world it was crooked."

Allow Others To Limit Their Potential

Especially as women, we receive criticism about every single thing we do, and this can put us at a disadvantage. If we listen to how others identify us, we are allowing them to limit our potential. Some people may deem you as a low-achieving individual, but that does not mean it's true. Your potential isn't set based on the labels that are placed upon you. Don't be willing to surrender your potential to the belief of others.

We often believe that the restrictions we've experienced earlier in life are permanent or we've been told that we have limitations we don't actually have. Either way, these things keep us from reaching our true potential. A limiting environment can also hold you back. Many people think that whatever environment they grew up in is normal and they start to believe that way of life is the only choice available to them.

To increase your potential, you must remove the forces that are holding you back. For example, if you are a woman who is passionate about becoming a leader and were born in a small, conservative town that doesn't value women in leadership roles, you need to separate yourself from that town. Staying in an environment that does not align with your values and goals will keep you from learning and expanding your potential.

As soon as you become aware that your limitations are not real or that they are a leash you can cut yourself loose from, you can open the door to growth.

Blame Themselves When Something Goes Wrong

It's important to accept responsibility for a mistake you made, but too often we beat ourselves up too harshly for it. Self-blame is toxic for ourselves and for others around us. It also draws in more toxicity, like mistreatment. Women who blame themselves for things gone wrong tend to attract abusive, manipulative partners. Their openness to taking the blame unconsciously encourages others to blame them as well.

It's possible to acknowledge what you've done wrong without attacking your character in the process. For instance, reframe your thoughts from, "I'm a bad person," to "I made a bad choice." This is key to helping you learn from your errors while simultaneously deflecting unnecessary criticism to who you are as a person.

"Self-blame prevents you from changing the environment. It keeps you focused on trying to fix yourself, even when there's nothing within you that needs to be fixed."

Making a mistake does not make you a bad person. Not everything is your fault. Due to their upbringing, some people may have more of a tendency to place the blame on themselves. Be aware that sometimes your brain is whispering nasty little lies to you. It's not always giving you an accurate portrayal of the situation at hand. Give yourself a break and do what it takes to get out of the cycle, which is definitely easier said than done. Seeking professional help is always a positive thing, so don't count that out.

Stay Silent

Whether it's reporting an incident to the authorities or standing up to someone abusing their power, women are pressured to stay silent for fear of the consequences or the lack of them. Some women might also believe that their voice does not matter, but a woman's genuine input can be invaluable to the lives of others. In addition, maintaining silence allows harmful patterns to continue repeating over and over and enables whoever or whatever is producing them. Staying silent also drains you of your mental strength.

Mentally strong women do not stay silent when they notice that something seems out of place or is unfair. Of course, sometimes it's up to you to read the room and decide whether speaking up is right or not for all the parties involved. They call others out on their behavior, keep people in check, and create a voice for themselves to let their ideas and opinions be heard. Women who break their silence make the world a better and safer place for all women to live in.

Refuse To Reinvent Themselves

At a certain point and time in life, some women refuse to reinvent themselves because they think their time is up or they view it as a hopeless effort because as the saying goes, you can't teach an old dog new tricks. Despite this popular belief, it is never too late to reinvent yourself. Whether you are 30 years old or 60, there is always room for improvement. It just means that you are still growing!

As you mature, your personality, priorities, and values will shift, and if you don't move in that same direction, you'll be unhappy about the spot you're in. You do not want to be at the end of your life and have regrets about not doing what you wanted to do.

Reinventing yourself doesn't mean throwing away all that you've learned in the past. In fact, all of the decisions, failures, achievements, and struggles have molded you into the person you are today. Remember that reinvention does not just happen in the span of a day; it is the kind of process that takes one day at a time.

If something keeps gnawing at you, it might be time to consider exploring that option. Listen to your inner voice and act on it, carefully and methodically, of course. Make that career change or move across the country, just don't let anyone tell you that you're too old to do it!

Fail To Acknowledge Their Successes

It's no surprise that women are reluctant to speak loudly about their successes because it is likely deeply rooted in misogyny and the conditioning to believe that men achieving successes outside of parenthood is the norm. Women frequently reject compliments by passing the credit down to someone else or quickly deflecting praise and attention by immediately returning the compliment. Although it's super uplifting and benevolent of you to show your support for other women, there is a time and place for it. During a moment when you're being complimented and admired is not the time to make it all about someone else. It's time to embrace yourself.

"Women need to stop downplaying their success. So many women struggle to say, 'Thank you,' even when given a genuine compliment...And women often downplay their success to their own detriment—on LinkedIn, in their resumes, and in job interviews..."

Mentally strong women don't downplay their success, but they also don't obnoxiously brag about it either. Practice responding with a simple "Thank you" rather than run away from the compliment. It is essential to remember that as women, acknowledging our successes and accepting compliments are ways of empowering ourselves. With the odds already stacked against us, minimizing our achievements sets us back further. It's all a process of learning and unlearning. As you continue to work on this, you will be able to speak confidently about yourself and realize that you deserve to because you earned it.

At the end of the day, no matter who we are, we all struggle with our mental health–or at least one of these destructive habits Morin speaks on. Morin ends her TED Talk by asking us to consider what bad mental habits or destructive beliefs are holding you back. Moreover, what is one small step you could take right here and right now to take control back? All of us have something we can work on, and, as we've seen–it really only takes one small step to get you started. So, what are you waiting for? It is time to take back control of your mental health, your thoughts, and ultimately–the way you live your life.

THE VERYWELL MIND PODCAST WITH AMY MORIN

Amy Morin's podcast, Verywell Mind, is yet another resource you can turn to for receiving sound advice and guidance on building mental strength and improving the state of your emotional and psychological health. On the show, every Monday, Morin interviews inspirational speakers from all different walks of life, many of whom are well-known, high-profile figures. Guest speakers usually reveal their strategies on how to best navigate their way through the journey of life. Some of the speakers include: IT cosmetics founder Jamie Kern Lima, three-time NBA all-star Steve Francis, and cookbook author Danielle Walker. Despite the fact that these successful people are all from vastly different industries–makeup, basketball, cooking–they each have experienced mental health struggles and incidents where their mental strength has been compromised.

One of the most notable stories shared on the podcast is "How to Save Yourself With Bestselling Author Danielle Walker." The 45 minute interview discusses Danielle Walker's relationship with food, with medicine, and with her mental health.

DANIELLE WALKER'S STORY

Danielle Walker is the author and photographer of the New York Times bestselling cookbook "Against All Grain." She was diagnosed with an autoimmune disorder called ulcerative colitis at the young age of 22, just barely graduated from college. Ulcerative colitis is a chronic, inflammatory bowel disease that causes inflammation in the digestive tract.

Medical professionals told her that she could live a normal life and manage her illness with the prescribed medications. But this was not what she wound up experiencing. She experienced debilitating side effects that were ultimately dismissed by the doctors, along with regular flare ups that forced her to be hospitalized multiple times.

After five years of suffering and moving in and out of hospitals, she thought that there had to be another, more efficient way to alleviate the pain and so she began looking for her own solutions. Through a long and arduous process, Walker figured out what foods she could keep in her diet and what needed to be eliminated. After discovering what few foods she could eat, she felt like meals were not as tasty and enjoyable as they used to be, so she set out to create recipes that tasted good and followed her diet. Eventually, her recipes blew up. People were interested in improving their health and changing their diets for the better. Walker's blog led to the creation of a cookbook, which led to her becoming a best-selling author.

Walker confessed to Morin that her diagnosis caused her to feel grief over what she felt she was losing. The ideals and the vision she had for her life since she was a child crumbled to pieces after hearing about her diagnosis. She revealed her past worries over if she would be able to have kids and the loss of eating traditional foods. She had hopes of passing down the traditional family recipes, but it seemed that this would be impossible and that all was lost.

Walker also expressed her frustrations with the invisibility of her disease and her suffering. She explained that with autoimmune disorders, most times the sickness itself can be invisible to the outside eye. There were certain times where it was obvious she was sick: she would look pale, emaciated, and lose tremendous amounts of weight. During the occasions when she was out of the hospital, friends and other acquaintances who didn't know any better, waved away her concerns, saying that she looked perfectly healthy.

Advice From Danielle Walker

At the end of the interview, Amy Morin sums up Walker's advice into three main points. First, see if what other people are saying actually lines up with your experience. Also, remind yourself that you are the expert on yourself. Doctors told Walker that she was fine and that diet had nothing to do with her condition. She saw and felt otherwise. Their words did not match up with her experience. Despite what others were telling her, she was still willing to take matters into her own hands to try to improve her circumstances anyway.

Second, tell your inner circle what you are going through, even if they can't directly relate. Sometimes you're not really looking for advice, but rather, a listening ear. Having a supportive shoulder to lean on and someone to hear you out can be just as helpful and relieving as receiving advice. Walker mentioned how her illness would cause her to be tired and lack energy. In the beginning stages, she often felt the need to explain to everyone why she had to skip out on a dinner outing or stay home from her kid's Christmas recital. She didn't want to be perceived as lazy, rude, or a bad mom.

"I don't have to prove myself. I'm a good mom."

Danielle Walker, "Verywell Mind" (2021).

Walker realized later on that it is not necessary to prove yourself or justify why you are missing events. Not caring what people think can really help to save your energy and focus on improving your own health. As long as you inform the people you trust, and are close to about what's going on, you don't need to explain yourself to people on the outside, who might not care to understand or even believe you.

"I look internally and try to not care about what other people think—which is always easier said than done."

Danielle Walker, "Verywell Mind" (2021).

She now prioritizes sleep and rest. She even determined the amount of hours she needs for her body to be feeling well when she wakes up in the morning. Walker admitted that sometimes it's tough to stick to her regimen, but declared that it's okay to pass up on social invitations in order to do what's best for your body. For example, if her husband suggests watching a movie together at a somewhat late hour, Walker claims that she has to put her foot down and go to sleep instead to get her allotted hours.

When Morin asked Walker where people looking to alter their diets should start, Walker answered that they should begin with a 30-day plan, which brings us to the third and last point. Run experiments for 30 days to gauge how you feel, whether it's trying the newly prescribed medication from your doctor, jogging every day, or cutting out specific foods and ingredients. Observe how you feel and how you function while doing those things–if it's better, worse, or the same.

While traditional medicine didn't help Walker much, it is still important to listen to health professionals' recommendations. Take their suggestions with a grain of salt because it's most likely not a foolproof cure, but doing some research and exploring the reasons behind their recommendations can help you gain a better understanding on why they are prescribing a new medication or adjusting your treatment plan.

About Her Cookbook

Danielle Walker's cookbook features delectable paleo recipes designed to help others suffering from ailments similar to hers to continue to enjoy food. Omitting grains, gluten, dairy, and refined sugars from your diet can make food boring and bland, but Walker combats this with "Against All Grain."

"Good times can still be had by those following the Paleo lifestyle."

Danielle Walker, "Against All Grain."

The paleo diet, also called the caveman diet or stone-age diet, is based on foods similar to what might have been eaten during the Paleolithic period, which dates all the way back to 2.5 million years ago. A paleo diet typically consists of foods that could be obtained from hunting and gathering, like for example, vegetables, nuts, seeds, fruits, fish, and lean meats. It avoids foods that arose in popularity when farming practices emerged, such as grains, legumes, and dairy products.

Walker stated that she had never planned to become a cookbook author, and that her cookbook was written out of necessity. She wanted to break it down for people, recipes, mental health and all, so they wouldn't have to go through the same turmoil of figuring everything out on their own, like she did. Walker stresses that not one diet works for everyone, and that the most important thing to do is to listen to what your body is telling you. The recipes she invented are what works for her, but they may not work for everyone. Apparently though, they must have benefited a lot of people, since the cookbook has become a bestseller.

"We asked my audience to submit their testimonials about how food saved them. And we got a lot of mental health comments that I wouldn't have expected."

Danielle Walker, "Verywell Mind" (2021).

During her interview with Morin, Walker pointed out that her recipes did not only help people dealing with gut disease or other digestive issues. She also received emails from individuals she would never have expected to hear from. People with rheumatism, arthritis, psoriasis, anxiety, depression, etc. contacted her, detailing how the changes they made to their diet enhanced their moods or strengthened their joints.

The cookbook expands the options and provides alternatives to dishes that were once off-limits to people like her. Part of the adjustments she made to her new lifestyle required her to focus on what she can have rather than what she can't. She found that she constantly was being asked about all the foods she can't eat, but that list of restrictions can go on for miles. It was often overwhelming and discouraging to go over that seemingly infinite list, so she switched her mindset.

"Trying to focus on the good and the things that I can have rather than focusing on deprivation has helped me significantly."

Walker noted that food was not the only contributor to her flare ups. She learned that stress and a dip in mental health can also lead to flare ups. In the beginning, Walker was overly stressed about being accidentally exposed to foods that could cause her harm, whether at a friend's house for dinner or at a restaurant. The stress of possible exposure was something she had to learn to live with. There will always be some risk and obsessing over it will actually hurt your health more. The only thing you can do is to be mindful about what you are eating.

Walker's mental health would also go downhill when the anniversary of her daughter's death would come around. On June 24, 2014, about seven years ago, Walker and her husband lost their daughter Aila Jane to a fatal fetal defect called Osteogenesis Imperfecta, Type II. Walker noticed that the stress from experiencing an emotional time caused her disease to flare up. This is why she values counseling as a way to help regulate that stress.

Danielle Walker has gone through many difficult situations, but through it all, food has always been her savior. Walker has a memoir coming out in the fall called "Food Saved Me: My Journey of Finding Health and Hope Through the Power of Food." The book goes into detail about her illness, her healing journey, and it also offers hope to readers who feel doomed or trapped by sickness or life in general. You can pre-order the memoir on Amazon.

EPILOGUE

Amy Morin has spread her influence across the lives of so many people and through so many ways. She is constantly looking to share information and advice with others whether it's by way of her books, her podcast, or simple conversations with individuals. Her tips are beneficial to everyone for building mental strength, reframing patterns of thought, and improving mental health. Amy Morin is a shining example of how women can take back control of their lives. She is enlightening, empowering, and overall, a wonderful role model for women and girls everywhere.

www.ingramcontent.com/pod-product-compliance
Lightning Source LLC
Chambersburg PA
CBHW061534250726
48657CB00005B/2227